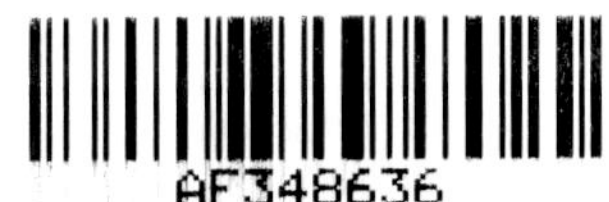


This Notebook Belongs To:

________________________________

Made in the USA
Monee, IL
07 July 2026

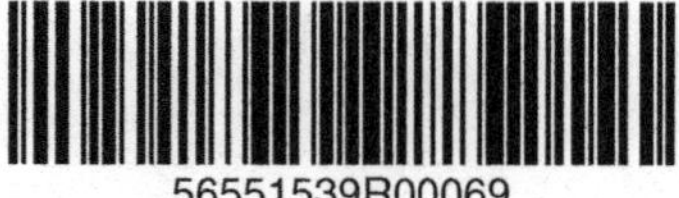

56551539R00069